DEFEATING MULTIPLE SCLEROSIS WITH EXPERT GUIDANCE

Ultimate Solution Handbook For Patients, Guardians Or Family To Understand, Manage, Treat, Prevent, Reverse Symptoms And Live Well

DR. POTTER WHITLEY

Copyright © 2023 by Dr. Potter Whitley

approval or validation is not implied by the inclusion of these references.

Any direct, indirect, incidental, special, or consequential damages resulting from using or not being able to use the material in this book are not covered by the author's liability policy. For medical advice and counsel particular to their circumstances, readers are advised to check with experienced healthcare specialists.

The content, materials, and information in this book are subject to change at any time without prior notice, at the author's discretion. The text may contain errors or omissions for which the author is not responsible.

By reading this book, you understand and accept the conditions of this disclaimer.

THE REASON BEHIND THIS BOOK

"Defeating Multiple Sclerosis With Expert Guidance" is a valuable resource for anyone traversing the complex terrain of Multiple Sclerosis (MS). It offers knowledge and empowerment. The first half of this thorough book starts with a fundamental investigation that dispels the myths surrounding MS and explores its different forms, possible causes, and the crucial elements of symptom recognition and diagnosis. By promoting a thorough comprehension of the illness, readers are better equipped to start along the path to efficient treatment and rehabilitation.

This book takes a comprehensive approach, delving deeper than the fundamentals and engrossing readers in the complex web of medical procedures. The second segment offers a road map through the medical complexities, from the variety of medical specialists involved in MS care to state-of-the-art diagnostic tests and novel medicines. With this information, readers can collaborate on their treatment plan by actively interacting with their healthcare team.

The third portion, which addresses the critical roles of nutrition, exercise, stress management, and quality sleep, is a goldmine for anyone looking to lead a balanced lifestyle while coping with the problems of multiple sclerosis. It highlights the transformational potential of lifestyle choices. Readers are encouraged to investigate a comprehensive road to MS care by fusing conventional medical procedures with holistic techniques, which promotes a sense of control over their well-being.

Most importantly, the guide acknowledges the value of having a strong support system during the MS journey. An insightful examination of the roles played by friends and family, the value of support groups, and the advantages of professional therapy are used in the fifth section to reveal the emotional support that people and their loved ones require.

The sections that follow guide readers through issues of everyday living, educational empowerment, and specific issues like women's health and pediatric MS.

This book is noteworthy for its forward-thinking approach, as it explores cutting-edge research topics and provides insights on advances, genetic influences, personalized medicine, and future directions in MS care.

Incorporating true success stories and motivational travels, which highlight the tenacity and victory of MS warriors, adds a touching touch. Readers are encouraged and motivated by these stories, which gives them hope and inspiration for their special journey.

"Defeating Multiple Sclerosis With Expert Guidance" is more than just a book; it is a source of inspiration, a road map for comprehension, and a handbook for people navigating the challenging landscape of multiple sclerosis. It helps individuals in need by providing not just knowledge but also a helping hand as they work to overcome the obstacles this condition presents.

TABLE OF CONTENT

[11]

CHAPTER ONE

UNDERSTANDING MULTIPLE SCLEROSIS
What Is The Definition Of Multiple Sclerosis?

A neurological disease that affects the brain and spinal cord collectively known as the central nervous system, multiple sclerosis (MS) is a chronic and sometimes fatal illness. In multiple sclerosis (MS), the immune system misinterprets the myelin sheath that protects nerve fibers, leading to impaired brain-to-body communication. It is currently unclear exactly what triggers this immune system failure in MS patients, which makes the illness difficult to treat and extremely complicated.

The growth of lesions or scars on the impacted nerve fibers is one of the characteristics of multiple sclerosis. Numerous symptoms are brought on by these lesions, which interfere with the normal passage of electrical impulses along the nerves. Multiple sclerosis (MS) is a heterogeneous disease because individual differences in the disease's severity and course occur. While some people may only have minor symptoms, others may be more severely disabled.

MS is more common in women than in males, and it typically manifests in early adulthood. With phases of relapse and remission, during which symptoms get worse before getting better, the disease's course can be unpredictable. Certain MS patients experience gradual progression without a noticeable remission, which over time might result in cumulative impairment. To effectively manage and treat multiple sclerosis, one must have a thorough understanding of the disease's nature.

Different Types and Forms of Multiple Sclerosis

There are several ways that multiple sclerosis manifests itself, and each has unique traits and progression patterns. Relapsing-remitting MS (RRMS), progressive-relapsing MS (PRMS), secondary progressive MS (SPMS), and primary progressive MS (PPMS) are the most prevalent forms.

Periods of symptom flare-ups (relapses) interspersed with partial or total recovery (remission) are the hallmarks of RRMS. As of the time of diagnosis, this is the most prevalent type of MS. With PPMS, symptoms develop gradually over time without noticeable relapses or remissions.

After an initial period of relapsing-remitting symptoms, SPMS usually progresses toward impairment more gradually. The least prevalent kind, PRMS, is characterized by a progressive course of symptoms interspersed with sporadic relapses.

It is critical to identify the precise type of MS a patient has to customize treatment regimens and forecast the disease's expected trajectory. For the best possible patient outcomes, tailored and targeted therapeutic approaches are essential, as each variant presents different obstacles and considerations.

Reasons and Danger Elements

Although the precise etiology of multiple sclerosis is still unknown, scientists think that a mix of environmental and genetic variables have a role in the disease's development. People with a family history of MS have a marginally increased chance of getting the disease, suggesting a genetic predisposition. But most cases cannot be explained by genetics alone, suggesting that environmental factors also matter a great deal.

Smoking, exposure to specific infections, and vitamin D insufficiency are environmental factors that have been researched about multiple sclerosis. Epstein-Barr virus infections, in particular, have been investigated for possible connections to the development of multiple sclerosis (MS). Vitamin D, which is obtained from sunlight and dietary sources, has been implicated in modulating the immune system and its deficiency has been associated with an increased risk of MS. Furthermore, it has been determined that smoking is a modifiable risk factor that could influence the development of MS as well as its course.

Untangling the complex web of factors that lead to the development of multiple sclerosis (MS) requires an understanding of the interplay between genetic susceptibility and environmental triggers. Research in this area is critical to identifying potential preventive strategies and more focused treatment options.

Signs and Prognosis

Numerous symptoms, such as exhaustion, trouble walking, tingling or numbness, weakening of the muscles, issues with coordination, and cognitive impairment, might be signs of multiple sclerosis. These symptoms are brought on by damage to the myelin sheath, which interferes with the brain's ability to communicate with other regions of the body. The difficulty of diagnosing multiple sclerosis is increased by the unpredictability of symptom onset and progression.

A variety of diagnostic tests, clinical assessment, and medical history analysis are frequently used in the diagnosis of multiple sclerosis. As a visual representation of the harm being done to the brain and spinal cord, magnetic resonance imaging, or MRI, is a vital tool in the detection of lesions in the central nervous system. Examining the fluid surrounding the brain and spinal cord is known as cerebrospinal fluid analysis, and it can be used to find particular anomalies that point to multiple sclerosis.

The difficult part of the diagnostic process is ruling out other disorders that have comparable symptoms to MS because there isn't a single, conclusive test for the disease. Additionally, there may be delays in diagnosis due to the diverse and unexpected character of MS symptoms. Initiating suitable treatment and symptom management strategies requires an early and accurate diagnosis, underscoring the significance of continuous research aimed at improving diagnostic instruments and techniques.

In summary, multiple sclerosis is a neurological disorder with a wide range of manifestations that are intricate and varied. As research into the disease's underlying mechanisms continues, hope for more targeted therapies and eventually a cure is offered. Developing effective treatment strategies and improving the quality of life for individuals living with MS requires an understanding of the disease's complexities, types, potential causes, and diagnostic challenges.

CHAPTER TWO

GETTING AROUND THE MEDICAL SYSTEM
Medical Experts Associated with MS Care:

A multidisciplinary team of medical specialists must work together to navigate the challenging terrain of Multiple Sclerosis (MS). Neurologists are the leaders in MS care, using their particular skills to identify and treat the illness. To create individualized treatment programs, these professionals evaluate the symptoms of their patients, perform neurological exams, and interpret diagnostic testing.

Nurses are also essential in monitoring for possible adverse effects, administering medication, and educating patients. The services of physical and occupational therapists are essential for improving patients' quality of life, taking care of mobility problems, and creating adaptable plans to deal with day-to-day obstacles. Psychologists and other mental health providers make a substantial contribution by addressing the psychological and emotional components of managing a chronic illness and providing support and coping mechanisms.

Additionally, due to the systemic nature of the disease, MS management frequently entails cooperation with experts like urologists, ophthalmologists, and rehabilitation specialists.

Urologists treat bladder dysfunction, a prevalent MS symptom, whereas ophthalmologists treat vision problems. Rehabilitation experts assist in creating workout plans that are suited to each person's capabilities, promoting self-sufficiency, and slowing the advancement of disabilities. Because of their combined expertise, MS care is provided in a comprehensive manner that recognizes the disease's complexity and customizes interventions to meet the individual needs of each patient.

Imaging And Diagnostic Tests:

Modern diagnostic testing and imaging methods are critical to the quick and accurate diagnosis of multiple sclerosis. To establish a preliminary diagnosis, neurologists utilize a range of diagnostic tools, including laboratory tests, clinical assessments, and medical history analysis. A vital component of diagnosis is Magnetic Resonance Imaging (MRI), which offers precise pictures of the brain and spinal cord. With contrast-enhanced MRI scans, lesions or regions of demyelination, which are diagnostic of multiple sclerosis, can be seen, helping to confirm the diagnosis.

A lumbar puncture allows for the examination of cerebral spinal fluid, which helps to detect specific markers associated with multiple sclerosis. Other diagnostic tools include evoked potential testing, which measures electrical activity in reaction to stimuli. Having these diagnostic instruments integrated makes it possible to comprehend the condition more thoroughly and accurately, which makes it easier to create individualized treatment regimens. Crucially, developments in imaging technologies keep improving diagnostic accuracy, allowing for earlier therapies and better results for MS patients.

Medications and Treatment Options:

Fighting Multiple Sclerosis requires a sophisticated strategy of care that makes use of a range of individualized choices. The mainstay of MS treatment is the use of illness-modifying Therapies (DMTs), which attempt to change how the illness progresses, lessen the frequency of relapses, and relieve symptoms. These drugs, which can be taken orally, intravenously, or as infusions, work by targeting the immune system to stop it from attacking the central nervous system.

Treatments for specific symptoms of multiple sclerosis (MS), such as fatigue, discomfort, and bladder dysfunction, are critical to their management. In addition to pharmaceutical interventions, physical and occupational therapy supports mobility, independence, and general well-being. Healthy eating, frequent exercise, stress reduction, and other lifestyle changes are all part of an all-encompassing approach to MS therapy that aims to improve patients' quality of life.

To customize interventions to each patient's specific requirements and preferences, healthcare providers work closely with individuals who have multiple sclerosis (MS). Patient input in treatment decisions is crucial. Consistent monitoring and modifications to treatment regimens guarantee sustained effectiveness and tackle any new obstacles, underscoring the dynamic aspect of managing multiple sclerosis.

New Research and Therapies:

The field of multiple sclerosis is always changing because of discoveries being made and advances in treatment. With the goals of increased convenience, decreased side effects, and increased efficacy, emerging medicines could offer MS patients more options. For example, monoclonal antibodies are a state-of-the-art research tool that precisely modulates the immune system by targeting specific components of the system.

The potential for stem cell therapy to regenerate injured nerve cells and restore function is being investigated. Personalized medicine approaches that take into account individual variability in treatment responses are made possible by research endeavors that also aim to understand the genetic and environmental factors that influence MS susceptibility. These approaches, though still in the experimental stages, highlight the scientific community's commitment to pushing the boundaries of treatment possibilities for the disease.

Clinical trials are essential to the advancement of MS research because they offer a framework for assessing new treatments and improving those that already exist. The success of these trials depends on the cooperation of researchers, medical experts, and people with MS. This ensures that the interventions are in line with the needs and difficulties that exist in the real world. There is optimism for a future where the effects of MS are further reduced as more targeted, efficient, and individualized medicines become possible as the scientific community works to understand the complexities of MS.

CHAPTER THREE

MS MANAGEMENT AND LIFESTYLE
Diet's Part in MS Management

The management of Multiple Sclerosis (MS), a chronic autoimmune illness affecting the central nervous system, is heavily influenced by diet. Even though there is no known cure for multiple sclerosis, following a nutritious and well-balanced diet helps slow the disease's course and enhance general well-being.

Studies indicate that specific food regimens may aid in the management of symptoms and improve the quality of life for people with multiple sclerosis.

The significance of an anti-inflammatory diet is one important factor. Omega-3 fatty acids, antioxidants, and anti-inflammatory foods can help reduce inflammation in the central nervous system, which is a defining feature of multiple sclerosis (MS). Include fatty fish, like salmon and mackerel, in your diet, as well as colorful fruits and vegetables.

Additionally, supporting brain health depends on keeping the right ratio of key minerals, such as vitamins B12 and D.

Certain diets, including the Mediterranean or low-saturated-fat diet, also help certain MS patients. By emphasizing whole foods, lean proteins, and healthy fats, these diets may improve cardiovascular health and lessen the intensity of MS symptoms.

Since the effects of diet can differ from person to person, people with MS must collaborate closely with nutritionists and medical professionals to customize their diet to meet their unique needs.

To sum up, a personalized and well-planned diet can be an effective management tool for multiple sclerosis (MS). By selecting foods that promote overall health and anti-inflammatory processes, people with MS can actively improve their quality of life and possibly slow down the disease's progression.

Physical Activity And Exercise:

Physical activity and exercise are essential for managing multiple sclerosis (MS). Exercise has been demonstrated to provide multiple advantages for people with MS, including better mobility and increased mental well-being, despite potential obstacles arising from the nature of the condition.

Muscle weakness, spasticity, and balance problems are just a few of the unique concerns that can be addressed with a customized fitness program for multiple sclerosis. Exercises focusing on strength training help strengthen weaker muscles and boost their tone and functionality. Aerobic activities, like swimming or walking, can support cardiovascular health and help reduce fatigue, a typical MS symptom.

Beyond its physical advantages, regular exercise has been associated with improvements in mood and cognitive function—two areas that MS can affect. The natural mood enhancer that is endorphin released during exercise can help people cope with the stress and depression that come with dealing with a chronic illness.

People with MS must collaborate closely with fitness specialists and medical professionals to create a personalized exercise regimen that fits their needs and limits. As the illness worsens, routine monitoring and modifications to the exercise regimen could be required.

In summary, adding exercise to one's daily regimen is a proactive and powerful way to manage multiple sclerosis (MS). It not only helps with physical limits but also has a good impact on mental and emotional health, which enhances one's quality of life overall.

Techniques for Stress Management:

One important component that might worsen Multiple Sclerosis (MS) symptoms and increase the disease's overall burden is stress. Therefore, to improve their well-being and maybe lessen the negative effects of stress on their condition, people with MS must learn efficient stress management skills.

For people with multiple sclerosis (MS), mindfulness and meditation are effective strategies for managing stress because they emphasize being in the present moment and minimizing worry about the past or the future. To assist people in developing resilience and an optimistic outlook, mindfulness can be especially helpful in addressing the emotional difficulties that frequently accompany a chronic illness.

Progressive muscle relaxation, which entails tensing and then gradually relaxing various muscle groups to encourage both physical and mental calm, is another useful stress-reduction method. For those with MS who may have tightness and stiffness in their muscles, this can be especially beneficial.

Another essential component of stress management is social support. Developing relationships with people who comprehend the difficulties of having Multiple Sclerosis (MS) helps foster a sense of belonging and lessen feelings of loneliness. Online and in-person support groups provide a forum for people to exchange experiences, coping mechanisms, and emotional support.

Acknowledging one's triggers and building a toolkit of coping skills are crucial. To effectively manage daily stressors, this may involve engaging in joyful activities, such as hobbies or creative endeavors, as well as establishing reasonable expectations and boundaries.

In conclusion, stress management is essential to controlling multiple sclerosis. People with Multiple Sclerosis (MS) can improve their overall quality of life and empower themselves to manage the emotional difficulties of the condition by implementing tailored coping strategies, mindfulness, relaxation techniques, and social support.

Sleep and Multiple Sclerosis:

Good sleep is essential for good health in general and should not be undervalued in terms of how it affects MS management. Sleep difficulties such as insomnia, fragmented sleep, and restless legs syndrome are common in people with multiple sclerosis (MS), and they can hurt their overall health and make their symptoms worse.

Resolving sleep problems is critical to successful MS management. Better sleep quality can be achieved by establishing a regular sleep schedule that helps the body's internal clock to be regulated. This entails keeping a consistent sleep routine, furnishing a cozy sleeping space, and engaging in relaxation exercises before going to bed.

Studies indicate a reciprocal association between sleep and symptoms of multiple sclerosis. Prioritizing sleep hygiene becomes an essential part of comprehensive MS management because, although MS-related symptoms can interfere with sleep, poor quality sleep can also lead to increased fatigue, impaired cognitive function, and heightened pain sensitivity—common challenges faced by individuals with MS.

In certain situations, medical interventions—such as drugs or therapies meant to address sleep disturbances—might be advised. However, making lifestyle changes and implementing sound sleeping practices can frequently result in notable gains. A more pleasant night's sleep can be achieved by avoiding stimulants close to bedtime, minimizing screen time before bed, and partaking in relaxing activities.

People with MS must be honest with medical practitioners about their sleep habits and any difficulties they may be having. As part of a comprehensive MS care plan, addressing sleep issues can improve daily functioning, improve symptom management, and improve quality of life overall.

In summary, understanding the complex connection between sleep and MS is essential for efficient treatment. People with MS can improve their general health and well-being and provide a stronger basis for managing the complications of the condition by emphasizing good sleep hygiene and seeking appropriate therapies when necessary.

CHAPTER FOUR

MULTIDISCIPLINARY METHODS FOR MS
Alternative & Complementary Medicine:

The comprehensive approach to managing Multiple Sclerosis (MS) includes a large component of Complementary and Alternative Medicine (CAM). As an alternative to conventional treatments, complementary and alternative medicine (CAM) aims to address the physical, mental, and emotional aspects of multiple sclerosis (MS). Therapies and practices that fall under the CAM umbrella include herbal supplements, dietary modifications, and various mind-body interventions.

The emphasis on individualized treatment is one noteworthy feature of CAM in MS management. CAM professionals frequently customize treatment programs based on each patient's unique constitution, lifestyle, and preferences. This customized approach acknowledges the wide range of patient responses to therapies as well as the intrinsic heterogeneity in MS symptoms. People with MS may benefit from a more thorough and customized approach to controlling their condition if complementary and alternative medicine (CAM) is included in the treatment plan.

Additionally, CAM methods frequently place a high priority on lifestyle changes and preventative actions, which support resilience and long-term health. This proactive approach is especially important for MS patients, as controlling the disease's development is critical. Patients get a sense of empowerment and self-efficacy when they investigate complementary therapies since they are equipped with new tools to actively engage in their health journey.

Mind-Body Techniques: Meditation and Yoga:

Mind-body therapies, like yoga and meditation, are essential components of integrative MS management strategies. These methods provide people with MS with a comprehensive approach to treating both physical symptoms and mental well-being since they acknowledge the connection between the mind and body.

Yoga is very beneficial for people with Multiple Sclerosis (MS). It helps with flexibility, balance, and strength and helps with some of the physical issues associated with the disease. It emphasizes gentle movements, stretching, and controlled breathing. Yoga's meditative elements also aid in stress reduction, which is important for controlling MS symptoms because stress can make the illness worse.

Another essential component of mind-body therapies is meditation, which gives people with MS an effective tool for building mental toughness. Particularly mindfulness meditation helps people learn to live in the present moment without passing judgment, which promotes emotional equilibrium and lessens anxiety related to the unknowns of having multiple sclerosis. Research has shown that consistent meditation practice may have a beneficial effect on the structure and function of the brain, which may have an impact on how the disease progresses.

Yoga and meditation develop a sense of agency and self-awareness in people, enabling them to take an active role in their healing process. These methods support the emotional and psychological health of MS patients as well as the physical components of the disease's management when used holistically.

MS and Acupuncture:

The traditional Chinese medical practice of acupuncture has received acceptance as an adjunctive treatment in the comprehensive care of multiple sclerosis (MS). This traditional method entails inserting tiny needles into predetermined bodily locations to encourage energy flow and systemic equilibrium. Acupuncture is thought to affect the immune system, lessen inflammation, and ease symptoms in the context of multiple sclerosis.

Acupuncture's ability to alleviate the neuropathic pain that many MS patients feel is one of its main advantages; research indicates that acupuncture may alter pain perception pathways, offering respite to people suffering from the chronic pain that comes with the disease. Acupuncture's effect on fatigue, a common MS symptom, has also been studied; preliminary results show improvements in energy and general well-being.

As an integrative and personalized approach to healthcare, acupuncture complements conventional treatments by addressing both physical symptoms and underlying imbalances. This holistic nature of acupuncture is in line with the comprehensive approach required for managing the multifaceted challenges of multiple sclerosis.

To guarantee a coherent and well-coordinated treatment plan, people with MS must collaborate with their healthcare team, just like they would with any supplemental therapy. When carefully integrated into the entire care plan, acupuncture can help manage multiple sclerosis (MS) holistically, improving overall health and quality of life.

Combining Conventional Treatments with Holistic Approaches:

A progressive and patient-centered approach to controlling Multiple Sclerosis (MS) involves the merging of holistic therapies with conventional therapy. Although traditional therapy, including disease-modifying medications, concentrates on altering the progression of the illness and controlling particular symptoms, integrative methods cover a wider range of interventions that attend to the total health of MS patients.

Collaboration and communication between practitioners of complementary and alternative therapies and healthcare professionals with expertise in traditional medicine is a crucial component of this integration. By starting an open discussion, one may make sure that all facets of a patient's health are taken into account and that treatment plans are coordinated to prevent duplication or disputes. This cooperative strategy aims to maximize the advantages for the MS patient while acknowledging the importance of each modality.

Furthermore, a more individualized and patient-centered treatment plan is made possible by the combination of holistic techniques. Since every person experiences MS differently, combining traditional and holistic treatments allows for a customized approach that takes into account each patient's particular needs and preferences. In addition to increasing treatment efficacy, this individualized care raises the patient's sense of autonomy and involvement in their health journey.

A more thorough understanding of the variables influencing MS, such as lifestyle, stress levels, and general mental health, can be achieved by incorporating holistic techniques. Complementary therapies, diet plans, and mind-body techniques may enhance the benefits of traditional treatments by providing extra resources for managing symptoms and enhancing the general quality of life for MS patients.

In summary, a progressive paradigm in MS management is the combination of traditional treatments with holistic techniques. Healthcare professionals can provide patients with MS with a more comprehensive, individualized, and empowered way to manage the challenges of having this chronic illness by fusing the advantages of both methods.

CHAPTER FIVE

ESTABLISHING A HELPFUL NETWORK
The Role of Friends and Family in MS Care:

The support of friends and family is crucial in the fight against Multiple Sclerosis (MS). MS has a significant effect on the person who has been diagnosed as well as their immediate support network. A supportive network is essential due to the condition's physical and mental toll. Friends and family can become strongholds, providing both emotional and practical support.

Family and close friends are invaluable in helping with everyday tasks that might be difficult for an individual with multiple sclerosis. Their assistance is necessary to keep things feeling normal, whether it's with domestic chores or getting to and from doctor's visits.

Furthermore, the existence of a supportive network is vital because the unpredictable nature of symptoms and the chronic nature of the disease can contribute to feelings of loneliness and sadness. The emotional support provided by loved ones also helps to battle the psychological obstacles connected with MS.

Open communication is essential, though, for the person with MS as well as for their loved ones. It is essential to comprehend one another's wants and difficulties to create a helpful atmosphere. It's also critical for friends and family to become educated on MS for them to understand its intricacies and be able to help their loved ones with greater knowledge and empathy.

Accessing Microsoft Support Groups:

Making connections with people who have gone through similar things is essential to creating a supporting network. MS support groups are fantastic places for people to connect, exchange stories, and learn how to deal with the difficulties that come with having the disease.

Becoming a member of these clubs promotes a shared understanding that goes beyond what family and friends can supply, in addition to giving one a sense of community.

People with MS can share personal experiences, talk about the newest therapy options, and trade helpful symptom management advice in support groups. This common understanding can give one a sense of empowerment and control over their condition. Moreover, these associations frequently plan occasions and undertakings that encourage an optimistic and dynamic way of living, stressing the significance of preserving both physical and mental health.

Individuals can also get assistance navigating the emotional components of MS by joining support groups. The sensation of loneliness that frequently accompanies chronic illnesses can be lessened by discussing worries, disappointments, and accomplishments with people who genuinely understand.

These support groups, which provide knowledge and a strong sense of camaraderie that is crucial in the fight against Multiple Sclerosis, essentially become a lifeline.

Expert Guidance and Support for Mental Health:

Living with multiple sclerosis (MS) can have a significant psychological impact, making professional counseling and mental health support an essential part of the wider network of treatment. Anxiety, worry, and grief are just a few of the many feelings that can surface after receiving an MS diagnosis. It takes specialist support to deal with these feelings, and professional therapy can offer the strategies required to manage the mental health issues related to multiple sclerosis.

An individual's mental health and sense of self-worth can be greatly affected by MS. Developing coping mechanisms and resilience is a necessary part of adjusting to a new normal when dealing with a chronic disease. Professional counselors can help. Additionally, mental health care can help ease the strains on family dynamics and relationships by providing a safe space for people to talk about their worries and fears.

Burnout among caregivers is another issue that is addressed as part of the professional therapy component. Supporting friends and family members may become more stressed and emotionally exhausted. Caregivers can continue to effectively support others while maintaining their mental health by receiving professional counseling and learning the required skills.

<u>Managing Interactions with MS:</u>

Building a supportive network requires understanding the intricacies of personal relationships, which might be impacted by multiple sclerosis. To make sure that relationships endure the difficulties brought on by the illness, communication is essential.

Empathy and understanding can be fostered by having candid discussions about how MS affects both parties.

MS may cause adjustments to daily routines and intimacy in relationships. It takes perseverance and a readiness to adjust to navigate through these changes. Couples counseling can offer a secure setting for discussing worries, anxieties, and expectations, enabling the partnership to develop and prosper despite obstacles.

Friends who are knowledgeable about multiple sclerosis (MS) can provide invaluable support and understanding, but maintaining connections in friendships may require modifications as social activities and plans may need to be adjusted to fit the needs of someone with the condition. It's important to communicate clearly about personal needs and boundaries to maintain partnerships that are meaningful and beneficial for all parties.

Managing relationships with MS in the workplace is also necessary. It could be necessary to educate coworkers and employers about the disease to foster a more understanding and accommodating work environment. A more encouraging professional network can be created by establishing open lines of contact and looking into workplace accommodations.

Essentially, managing relationships with multiple sclerosis (MS) requires constant communication, knowledge, and a mutual resolve to adjust and assist each other during the condition's several phases. Developing resilient ties becomes essential to the larger network that aims to eradicate Multiple Sclerosis.

CHAPTER SIX

OVERCOMING DAY-TO-DAY DIFFICULTIES
Handling Tiredness and Mental Problems

Fatigue and cognitive problems are two of the many difficulties that come with having Multiple Sclerosis (MS). A common description of fatigue in multiple sclerosis is extreme tiredness that is not always alleviated by rest. A multifaceted approach is needed to effectively manage fatigue, including lifestyle modifications, energy-saving techniques, and good communication with healthcare providers. Getting regular, capacity-appropriate exercise, maintaining proper sleep hygiene, and controlling stress can all help reduce weariness.

For people with multiple sclerosis (MS), cognitive problems—such as memory loss, attention problems, and information processing difficulties—can have a substantial influence on day-to-day functioning. Cognitive rehabilitation, which entails a variety of cognitive exercises and methods, has demonstrated promise in reducing these difficulties. People with MS can also benefit from employing memory aids, planning their daily duties, and asking loved ones for support. A supportive work environment can be facilitated by having open communication regarding cognitive challenges with coworkers and employers.

People with MS must actively look for ways to improve their general well-being while still being aware of and accepting of their limits. Fatigue and cognitive difficulties can be effectively handled with appropriate coping skills, enabling people with MS to enjoy satisfying lives.

Modifications to the Home and Accessibility

To preserve their independence and quality of life, people with MS must live in an accessible environment. Making changes to your home is essential to reaching this objective. Easy modifications, like adding grab bars to restrooms and wheelchair-accessible ramps, can greatly improve mobility and safety. Accessibility is improved with lowered counters, broader entrances, and longer hallways.

Making inclusive changes that take into account each person's particular requirements is just as important as making structural adjustments when it comes to adapting to the home environment. This may include moving furniture around to make the space simpler to navigate or utilizing smart home technologies to regulate different elements of the living space. Working together with occupational therapists can yield insightful information on tailored adjustments that take into account each person's strengths and challenges.

Accessibility is not limited to the house; it also includes public areas, transit, and places of employment. Promoting universal design and raising knowledge of accessibility requirements can help create a society that is more accepting of people with multiple sclerosis.

Financial and Employment Considerations

Managing the work environment while living with multiple sclerosis necessitates giving job and money matters some thought. It is a personal choice to disclose one's MS diagnosis to employers; this decision is frequently impacted by the type of work being done and the amount of support offered. Having open lines of communication with employers about flexible work schedules and possible adjustments is essential to a successful and long-lasting career.

Financial factors are taken into account because medical costs and possible job changes may affect a person's budget. To reduce financial stress, it is crucial to investigate insurance coverage, employment modifications, and disability benefits. Long-term planning becomes especially crucial, encompassing estate planning and retirement concerns.

Support systems from society at large as well as from the workplace are essential for overcoming obstacles related to jobs and money. Making connections with advocacy organizations and consulting experts in MS-related job matters can offer helpful direction.

Advice and Safety Measures for MS Travelers

When traveling, people with multiple sclerosis need to prepare ahead and take potential obstacles into account. Changes in routine, weariness, and mobility issues can all affect how enjoyable a trip is. Being well-prepared is essential, beginning with a detailed investigation of the accessibility and medical facilities of the selected location. Traveling can be made more enjoyable by choosing lodging with accessible amenities and close to medical facilities.

Travel schedules should be adaptable, allowing for breaks and changes in response to energy levels. It is important to include prescription drugs, medical records, and assistive technology. To ensure a comfortable travel experience, it is recommended to let accommodation providers and transportation providers know in advance about any special needs.

When traveling, staying hydrated, controlling stress, and using relaxation techniques can all help lessen the effects of multiple sclerosis. People with MS should prioritize self-care and be aware of their physical and mental well-being when traveling by air, land, or sea.

In conclusion, people with MS can not only manage everyday barriers but also lead meaningful and rewarding lives if they plan, communicate well, and take a proactive approach to problem-solving.

CHAPTER SEVEN

EMPOWERING YOURSELF THROUGH EDUCATION
Staying Informed about MS Research:

When it comes to fighting Multiple Sclerosis (MS), it's critical for those who want to educate themselves to become empowered to stay up to date on the most recent research findings. The field of MS research is always changing as discoveries provide light on possible breakthroughs, novel treatment approaches, and a better comprehension of the illness. People who are empowered arm themselves with information, allowing them to make better decisions regarding their health and available treatments.

Attending conferences, keeping up with scientific publications, and interacting with respectable MS organizations are all essential components of remaining educated. These platforms offer a multitude of information, ranging from newly developed therapy strategies to profound understandings of the fundamental mechanics behind the illness. Keeping up with the most recent discoveries and advancements in multiple sclerosis can be ensured by routinely reviewing updates from groups like the European Committee for Treatment and Research in Multiple Sclerosis or the National Multiple Sclerosis Society.

Furthermore, connecting with others going through similar struggles might be facilitated by participating in MS-specific online networks and forums. These online forums frequently function as central locations for exchanging firsthand treatment stories, debating the most recent scientific discoveries, and providing support. People who actively participate in these groups receive both information and emotional support, which strengthens their path toward empowerment.

Essentially, keeping up with MS research is an ongoing effort that calls for active involvement with a variety of information sources. By doing this, people not only help others become advocates for their health but also add to the body of information, creating a community that is united in its opposition to the difficulties presented by multiple sclerosis.

Knowing Clinical Trials:

Those who want to take charge of their fight against Multiple Sclerosis (MS) must have a thorough understanding of clinical trials. Clinical trials, which look into novel therapies, drugs, and treatment modalities, are the cornerstone of medical advancement. Gaining control over one's health and advancing MS research can be achieved by actively participating in and understanding the complexities of these trials.

Clinical trials are organized research projects intended to assess the effectiveness and safety of novel therapies or interventions. By actively taking part in these trials, people with MS can significantly influence how MS is managed in the future. Comprehending the several stages of clinical trials, ranging from preliminary examination to extensive research enables individuals to make knowledgeable choices regarding their involvement by balancing the potential advantages against potential hazards.

Gaining knowledge about clinical trials and their implications for daily life, as well as ethical issues and informed consent procedures, is a necessary step towards self-empowerment. It also necessitates gathering information from trustworthy sources, like medical experts, academic institutions, and MS-specific organizations. To help people understand the intricacies of clinical trials and make decisions that are in line with their health objectives, numerous organizations offer information.

In summary, having a solid grasp of clinical trials gives people the ability to take an active role in their healthcare journey, thereby empowering them. People can help in the search for more potent therapies and, eventually, a cure for multiple sclerosis by actively taking part in these studies or by lending support to those who do.

Promoting Ms Awareness:

One effective way to empower oneself and the larger MS community is to advocate for MS awareness. Since multiple sclerosis (MS) is a complicated and sometimes misdiagnosed condition, advocacy is essential in debunking myths, increasing public awareness, and creating a welcoming atmosphere for people who are impacted. Individuals with MS can have a long-lasting influence on public opinion, resource accessibility, and the general quality of life for MS patients by volunteering as advocates.

A key component of effective advocacy is elevating the voices of MS patients, sharing personal accounts, and busting myths about the illness. Numerous avenues, such as social media, neighborhood gatherings, and cooperation with MS advocacy groups, might be used to accomplish this. People can personalize the experiences of people with MS by actively engaging with the public, which will elicit empathy and understanding from a larger audience.

Another essential component of empowering oneself with MS knowledge is legislative advocacy. People can collaborate with advocacy groups to advocate for better access to healthcare services, more money for MS research, and the creation of laws that assist those with long-term illnesses. By actively engaging in advocacy initiatives, people help shape laws that directly affect the MS community and build a more accepting and inclusive social structure.

Additionally, supporting accessible workplace policies and surroundings enables people with MS to remain independent and make valuable contributions to their communities. In addition to helping the individual, this type of lobbying promotes a larger cultural movement in favor of tolerance and understanding.

To sum up, raising awareness of MS is a dynamic and comprehensive strategy for empowerment. Through promoting awareness, debunking misconceptions, and actively engaging in advocacy campaigns, individuals significantly contribute to the development of a more understanding and encouraging environment for those impacted by multiple sclerosis.

Resources for Patients and Caregivers to Learn:

By using a wide range of educational resources designed specifically for patients and caregivers, one can empower themselves by learning how to overcome Multiple Sclerosis. These resources are vital for comprehending the illness, figuring out available treatments, and creating a network of support. People can build a proactive approach to managing MS, broaden their knowledge base, and make well-informed decisions by actively seeking out and interacting with educational materials.

Many educational tools are available from reputable MS groups, including the Multiple Sclerosis International Federation and the National Multiple Sclerosis Society. These could include instructional booklets, webinars, online classes, and support groups covering a wide range of subjects, from MS research developments to symptom management. Through the utilization of these materials, people can acquire a thorough comprehension of the illness and all of its aspects.

Apart from official associations, virtual platforms, and discussion boards offer insightful perspectives derived from the real-life experiences of people with multiple sclerosis and their caregivers. Participating in these groups helps people learn from others going through similar struggles by fostering a sense of shared knowledge and support. Peer-to-peer learning turns into a potent empowerment tool since it offers real-world advice on how to handle day-to-day living with multiple sclerosis.

In the process of empowerment, education for caregivers is equally important. Resources that address the particular difficulties experienced by caregivers—such as mental health and useful caring techniques—help create a more complete support network. Armed with information, caregivers can help individuals with MS more successfully and foster a supportive environment for them.

To sum up, educational resources are essential for empowering people with multiple sclerosis and their caregivers. People can develop a foundation of knowledge that serves as the basis for self-advocacy, informed decision-making, and a proactive approach to managing the challenges of living with multiple sclerosis by actively engaging with these materials.

CHAPTER EIGHT

WOMEN'S HEALTH AND MS
MS and Pregnancy:

For women who have Multiple Sclerosis (MS), pregnancy can be a complicated and difficult time due to the interaction between autoimmune diseases and hormonal changes. The influence of pregnancy on the course of MS is one common feature. Interestingly, many women have a brief remission of symptoms during pregnancy, which is known as the "pregnancy effect." Hormonal changes, specifically elevated levels of progesterone and estrogen, are thought to have immunomodulatory effects during this period of remission.

Nonetheless, because there is an increased risk of recurrence during the postpartum period, it is imperative that women with MS exercise caution throughout pregnancy. The management of multiple sclerosis symptoms and the maintenance of a healthy pregnancy require close collaboration between neurologists and obstetricians to navigate the delicate balance. To reduce hazards to the growing fetus, it may be necessary to adapt certain disease-modifying medicines, making medication management an essential component.

Furthermore, it's important to recognize the psychological effects of pregnancy when dealing with multiple sclerosis. Women may struggle with worries about their capacity to raise a kid or worry about how MS may affect their experience as parents. It becomes critical during this phase to establish a strong support network that includes family, mental health professionals, and healthcare providers.

Hormonal Shifts with Symptoms of MS:

The complex association between hormonal fluctuations and multiple sclerosis symptoms complicates the disease's management even further, especially for women. The degree and frequency of MS symptoms have been linked to variations in estrogen levels, which can happen during the menstrual cycle, pregnancy, and menopause. Comprehending these dynamics is essential to customizing treatment plans and improving the general quality of life for female MS patients.

Personalized treatment plans that take hormonal influences into account are necessary because research indicates that hormonal fluctuations can affect immune responses and potentially impact the inflammatory processes associated with multiple sclerosis. Additionally, some women may experience an exacerbation of symptoms during specific phases of the menstrual cycle. This complex understanding emphasizes how crucial it is to use a multidisciplinary strategy to treat the interrelated elements at play holistically, integrating endocrinologists, gynecologists, and neurologists.

Furthermore, new treatments that focus on particular hormone pathways show promise for more accurate and successful MS symptom control. The goal of ongoing research is to disentangle the complex relationships between hormones and multiple sclerosis (MS), opening the door for novel treatments that take the individual's hormonal background into account.

Fertility and Family Planning Considerations:

Navigating the junction of reproductive decisions, disease management, and potential effects on the health of the mother and child is necessary for family planning for women with multiple sclerosis. The decision to have a family must be carefully considered in light of the special difficulties that MS presents, as well as the possible impacts that pregnancy and delivery may have on the progression of the illness.

Neurologists, reproductive experts, and obstetricians frequently work together to ensure optimal fertility and a successful pregnancy. Women who have multiple sclerosis (MS) may experience unique difficulties with reproduction, such as irregular menstruation or hormonal imbalances. To address these issues, a thorough evaluation of the person's reproductive health is required, along with the potential need for assisted reproductive technology.

Apart from fertility concerns, a crucial part of family planning for women with multiple sclerosis is ensuring the safety of disease-modifying therapies during conception and pregnancy. Certain medications have the potential to endanger the developing fetus, so a thorough assessment and possible modification of the treatment regimen are required. To make these difficult decisions, the woman, her partner, and her healthcare team must collaborate.

Preconception counseling also turns into a useful tool, giving MS women a chance to talk about their reproductive objectives, address any worries, and get personalized advice on how to best take care of their health before starting a family. With the development of assisted reproductive technologies and our increasing awareness of how multiple sclerosis affects fertility, it is essential to arm women with information and resources so they may make well-informed decisions about family planning.

Women-Focused Methods For Managing MS:

Women-centric approaches to managing Multiple Sclerosis (MS) are becoming more prevalent as a result of awareness of the distinctive features of the disease in females. Customizing therapies to meet the unique requirements and difficulties experienced by women with multiple sclerosis recognizes the impact of reproductive issues, hormonal changes, and general quality of life.

Customized treatment regimens that take into account a woman's hormonal fluctuations from adolescence through menopause are an essential component of a women-centric approach. More focused therapies are made possible by acknowledging the possible impact of hormonal changes on the intensity of symptoms and the course of the disease. To create comprehensive solutions that address the autoimmune nature of multiple sclerosis (MS) and the particularities of women's health, this strategy calls for close collaboration between neurologists, gynecologists, and other healthcare experts.

Moreover, comprehensive wellness programs are essential to women-focused MS management. Including dietary changes, physical activity, and mental health assistance in your lifestyle can have a positive effect on your general well-being. For example, it has been demonstrated that physical activity benefits people with multiple sclerosis in both psychological and physical ways. Certain exercises can help with concerns like exhaustion and balance, which are especially important for women.

Creating a community of support and offering tools to women who have multiple sclerosis can also help to build resilience and a sense of empowerment. Online discussion boards, peer support groups, and educational resources specific to women's experiences with multiple sclerosis can improve emotional health and increase awareness of the illness.

To sum up, adopting women-centric approaches to managing multiple sclerosis necessitates a thorough comprehension of the distinct obstacles encountered by women during their illness. Through the integration of medical expertise, individualized treatment regimens, and a holistic well-being emphasis, healthcare practitioners can enable women diagnosed with multiple sclerosis (MS) to confidently and resiliently traverse their distinct healthcare journey.

CHAPTER NINE

PARTICULAR CONSIDERATIONS FOR PEDIATRIC MS
Identifying and Classifying MS in Children:

Because pediatric multiple sclerosis (MS) is uncommon and shares symptoms with other childhood neurological disorders, it presents a special set of difficulties. Effective management requires early detection and precise diagnosis. A multidisciplinary approach integrating the knowledge of pediatricians, neurologists, and imaging specialists is necessary to recognize pediatric MS. Pediatric MS affects children and adolescents, in contrast to adult MS, which typically manifests between the ages of 20 and 40. As a result, healthcare providers must take age-appropriate symptoms into account.

A comprehensive medical history, a clinical examination, and the rule out of other possible causes are frequently the first steps in the diagnosis of pediatric MS. Neuroimaging is essential; magnetic resonance imaging (MRI) sheds light on the central nervous system lesions typical of multiple sclerosis (MS); nevertheless, interpreting these results in the context of juvenile development calls for specific knowledge. Cerebrospinal fluid analysis can also be used to find particular markers that point to multiple sclerosis.

Distinguishing MS symptoms from those of other pediatric conditions is a challenge. Numerous neurological symptoms, such as fatigue, balance problems, and cognitive impairment, can appear in children with multiple sclerosis. Accurate diagnosis requires a nuanced understanding of age-appropriate neurodevelopmental milestones. This highlights how important it is for parents, teachers, and medical professionals to work together to recognize early warning signs so that pediatric MS patients can receive timely intervention and experience better outcomes.

Treatment Strategies for MS in Children and Adolescents:

A customized strategy that takes into account the distinct physiological and psychological characteristics of kids and teenagers is needed to treat pediatric multiple sclerosis. Younger patients' disease progression has been effectively slowed by disease-modifying therapies (DMTs), which are frequently used in adult MS patients. However, the long-term effects on growth and development as well as any possible side effects must be carefully considered during the selection and administration of these therapies.

Comprehensive care for young MS patients encompasses physical, cognitive, and emotional aspects of their well-being in addition to pharmacological interventions. Occupational therapy, psychological support, and physical therapy are essential in addressing how the disease affects a child's day-to-day functioning and overall quality of life. Fostering an active partnership in the management of pediatric multiple sclerosis requires educating patients and their families about the disease, available treatment options, and potential lifestyle modifications.

Another crucial component of care is the change from pediatric to adult care. To guarantee the consistent application of treatment strategies and the tracking of the disease's progression, there needs to be a smooth transition of care that involves communication between pediatric and adult healthcare providers. Furthermore, continued research into cutting-edge therapeutic strategies tailored to pediatric MS patients has the potential to expand treatment options and enhance young patients' long-term outcomes.

Educational and Social Resources for Young MS Patients:

Pediatric MS has a profound effect on a child's social and educational development in addition to its effects on health. Comprehensive care for pediatric MS patients includes social and educational support because these settings help these young people with specific challenges that they face in their academic and social lives.

To ensure that children with MS can access and participate in learning activities effectively, educational accommodations are essential. These accommodations could take the form of specialized lesson plans, adjustments to the physical setting, and assistance from teachers who have been specially trained to meet the needs of students with long-term medical conditions. Implementing and maintaining these accommodations requires cooperation between parents, teachers, and medical professionals.

The obstacles presented by the disease have a significant impact on peer relationships, self-esteem, and emotional well-being. Social support is essential in reducing the psychosocial effects of pediatric MS. Online and in-person support groups offer pediatric MS patients invaluable forums for networking with like-minded individuals. Coping with the emotional aspects of having a chronic neurological condition can be made easier with the help of psychosocial interventions like counseling and cognitive-behavioral therapy.

Furthermore, encouraging knowledge and comprehension among peers, instructors, and school officials contributes to the development of a welcoming and encouraging atmosphere. For young MS patients, this creates a feeling of community, reducing the risk of social isolation and improving their general quality of life.

Prospects for the Future for Young MS Patients:

Young MS patients face a complex interplay of medical, psychological, and social factors that will determine their long-term prognosis. A comprehensive strategy that takes into account the changing needs of children and adolescents as they enter adulthood is necessary for comprehending and treating pediatric multiple sclerosis.

Improvements in pediatric MS medicine have led to a more promising prognosis in the long run. Current research efforts concentrate on improving treatment strategies, reducing adverse effects, and creating medications that are especially suited to the distinct features of the growing nervous system. There is hope for better results as our knowledge of the illness grows and we may be able to implement earlier interventions and more successful management techniques.

A smooth transition of care between pediatric and adult care requires careful planning and coordination between healthcare providers, patients, and families. This is a critical point in the long-term management of multiple sclerosis. To enable a smooth integration into adult healthcare systems, this transition entails attending to changing healthcare needs, factors related to education and employment, and psychosocial support.

Psychosocial factors are crucial in determining how young MS patients will fare in the long run. A positive self-image, coping mechanisms, and resilience-building are essential elements of psychosocial support. Young MS patients who have access to counseling services, support groups, and mental health resources are better able to deal with the emotional obstacles that may come up during their illness.

The changing face of pediatric MS care emphasizes how crucial it is for medical professionals, researchers, educators, and families to continue working together. By addressing the complex features of the illness, we open the door to a more optimistic prognosis in the long run and enable young people with MS to live happy, productive lives despite the obstacles their disease presents.

CHAPTER TEN

SOPHISTICATED SUBJECTS IN MS RESEARCH
Novel Findings in MS Research:

Recent years have seen ground-breaking advances in the study of multiple sclerosis (MS), giving patients new hope and changing our understanding of the condition. One important finding is the identification of particular immune system mechanisms that contribute to the progression of multiple sclerosis.

By delving deeply into the complex network of immune responses, scientists have identified important molecular pathways that underlie the immune system's erroneous attacks on the central nervous system. These discoveries open new avenues for targeted therapies that target and modulate these particular immune responses, in addition to providing light on the underlying causes of multiple sclerosis.

In addition, the field has made great progress toward creating disease-modifying therapies (DMTs) that are less harmful and have better efficacy. Research on biomarkers and advanced imaging technologies have made it possible to gain a more complex understanding of the course and activity of disease. These developments represent a paradigm shift in the treatment of multiple sclerosis (MS), shifting from symptom management to targeted interventions that attempt to change the course of the disease. This has led to the identification of novel drug targets, fostering the creation of medications that not only alleviate symptoms but also address the underlying pathology of MS.

In the field of neuroregeneration, another noteworthy development has occurred. From stem cell therapies to neuroprotective agents, researchers have investigated novel approaches to encourage the regeneration and repair of damaged nerve tissues in MS patients. These interventions hold promise in partially reversing the neurological damage caused by the disease. The potential for neuroregeneration provides a ray of hope for better functional outcomes and opens up new avenues for improving the quality of life for people with MS.

To sum up, the latest developments in MS research are revolutionary, providing hitherto unseen perspectives into the workings of the illness and possible treatment paths. These findings could lead to more individualized and successful treatment plans as the field develops, ultimately enhancing the lives of MS patients.

Environmental and Genetic Factors:

The disease known as multiple sclerosis (MS) is complicated and results from the intricate interaction of environmental and genetic factors. Investigating these factors has revealed a complex picture that has given important new information about susceptibility, the beginning and course of disease, and its progression. Numerous genetic variations linked to an increased risk of multiple sclerosis have been found through genetic studies, highlighting the polygenic nature of the illness. Genetics, however, affects more than just susceptibility; it also affects how a disease progresses and how well it responds to treatment.

Large-scale genomic studies made possible by the Human Genome Project and later cooperative efforts have enabled researchers to identify particular genetic variations associated with multiple sclerosis (MS).

Knowledge of the genetic basis of the disease not only helps predict risk but also provides opportunities for the development of personalized therapies based on individual genetic profiles. There is great potential for improving treatment outcomes and reducing side effects with this individualized approach.

The complex interaction between genetics and environment is evident in the way that people with a genetic predisposition may experience disease onset or exacerbation in the presence of specific environmental factors. On the environmental front, factors like smoking, vitamin D deficiency, and Epstein-Barr virus infection have emerged as potential triggers or exacerbators of MS.

Developing thorough preventative and intervention strategies requires dissecting these intricacies.

Furthermore, the significance of the microbiome in multiple sclerosis has come to light, emphasizing the complex interplay between immunological response and gut health.

Comprehending how the microbiome influences immune responses in multiple sclerosis opens up new possibilities for therapeutic interventions, possibly involving the modification of gut microbial communities.

In conclusion, research on the interaction between genetics and environment highlights how complex MS is. Untangling these subtleties will help develop a more sophisticated understanding of MS susceptibility, development, and treatment response as research advances, opening the door to individualized and focused therapy approaches.

MS and personalized medicine:

Treatment for multiple sclerosis (MS) has entered a new age with the development of personalized medicine, which offers individualized methods that take into account patient differences in genetics, environment, and disease characteristics. This paradigm change acknowledges the variety of MS and the fact that every patient's experience with the disease is different, marking a break from the conventional one-size-fits-all approach.

Genetic profiling is a crucial component of customized treatment in multiple sclerosis. Thanks to developments in genomics, scientists have been able to pinpoint particular genetic markers linked to MS susceptibility, disease progression, and responsiveness to treatment. By incorporating this genetic data into treatment choices, physicians can tailor therapy strategies to maximize effectiveness and reduce adverse effects. Medication choices made for patients based on their genetic profile may be advantageous, resulting in more specialized and focused care.

Personalized medicine in multiple sclerosis goes beyond genetics to include biomarkers and sophisticated imaging methods. Finding quantifiable markers that represent disease activity and therapy response is the goal of biomarker research. These indicators are useful tools for tracking the course of a disease and customizing therapy regimens to meet the needs of each patient. Furthermore, cutting-edge imaging technologies give medical professionals precise information about the degree of brain injury, which helps them make treatment decisions and promote early intervention.

In addition, the idea of "treating to target" has become more well-known in customized MS care. With this method, therapy plans are modified by the unique characteristics of each patient, and precise therapeutic goals are established. Through vigilant observation of disease activity and therapy response, physicians can modify therapies to conform to the distinct MS experience of each patient.

In summary, personalized medicine is a revolutionary method of treating multiple sclerosis (MS), utilizing genetic information, biomarkers, and sophisticated imaging to customize treatments based on patient needs. Better treatment outcomes and a higher quality of life for MS patients are anticipated as the field develops and customized medicine is incorporated into standard clinical practice.

Future Paths for MS Care and Treatment:

There are hopeful directions that could completely alter the way that multiple sclerosis (MS) is treated and cared for, and these changes are about to occur. With researchers delving into new therapy approaches and state-of-the-art technologies, the future of MS care seems bright and patient-focused.

The creation of precision medicines that target particular molecular pathways implicated in the pathophysiology of MS represents one encouraging avenue. The development of highly focused drugs with the ability to more successfully alter the course of the disease has been made possible by the identification of important immunological and neurodegenerative targets. With precision treatments, there is potential for more robust and long-lasting treatment effects as they target the fundamental mechanisms driving MS development in addition to symptom relief.

Research on neuroregeneration is also pointing to a bright future for MS patients: experimental treatments that encourage the regeneration and repair of injured nerve tissue may be able to partially restore some of the neurological impairments linked to the illness. Neuroprotective medications, stem cell therapies, and other cutting-edge methods provide a window into a time when functional recovery from MS becomes a feasible objective.

Furthermore, disease monitoring and management are about to undergo a revolutionary change thanks to the incorporation of artificial intelligence and digital health technology into MS care. Real-time tracking of symptoms, treatment responses, and lifestyle factors is made possible by wearable technology, smartphone applications, and data analytics platforms. This abundance of information enables more proactive and individualized approaches to MS care for both patients and healthcare professionals.

In conclusion, breakthroughs in precision medicine, neuroregeneration, and digital health technology are driving an unprecedented sense of hope for the treatment and care of MS patients in the future. The field of managing multiple sclerosis (MS) is expected to change as a result of these developments, providing new opportunities for better patient outcomes and a deeper comprehension of this intricate neurological condition.

CHAPTER ELEVEN

ACHIEVEMENTS AND MOTIVATIONAL TALES
Actual Life Recollections of MS Warriors

When it comes to fighting Multiple Sclerosis (MS), the firsthand accounts of these soldiers serve as potent monuments to the resilience of the human spirit. Every person's path is a distinct account of fortitude, bravery, and tenacity in the face of an arduous and unpredictably changing circumstance. MS patients frequently have to navigate a challenging array of symptoms, ranging from exhaustion and problems with movement to mental difficulties. Despite these extreme challenges, their tales demonstrate not only survival but also success in the face of hardship.

A lot of MS fighters remember the first shock of receiving the diagnosis, which changed their life and made them face the unknown. The resilience shown is nothing short of astounding, and both physical and emotional modifications are needed. These people have an amazing ability to adjust to the always-evolving nature of MS, altering their daily schedules and adopting novel symptom management techniques. MS warriors embody perseverance, from examining different treatment options to implementing lifestyle adjustments.

Furthermore, MS warriors' support systems can have a significant impact on their path. A strong base of support and comprehension is provided by friends, family, and medical experts. The relationships that develop inside these networks of support play a crucial role in the story as a whole, illustrating not only the strength of the individual but also the strength that comes from belonging to a community.

Along with taking on obstacles, these MS warriors are redefining the conventional narrative surrounding disability. To inspire others and debunk misconceptions about MS, many participate in advocacy and awareness campaigns. By sharing their personal stories, they empower others and create a feeling of community, transforming their problems into sources of hope for those who may be at an earlier stage of their MS journey.

MS fighters are shining examples of resiliency in the broad tapestry of real-life experiences; they personify the philosophy of meeting adversity head-on and coming out stronger on the other side. Their tales go beyond the confines of illness to become tales of inspiration, victory, and the resiliency of the human spirit.

Overcoming Adversity

In the context of Multiple Sclerosis (MS), triumphs over adversity are narratives of great human successes, resilience, and the unwavering pursuit of a fulfilling life rather than merely instances of overcoming physical problems. Multiple sclerosis (MS) poses significant challenges that require not just physical strength but also a persistent mindset due to its unpredictable nature and wide range of symptoms.

For many people with MS, the path consists of a constant stream of small and large victories. Getting over the initial shock of receiving a diagnosis and adjusting to a new normal could be the first steps. Overcoming hardships frequently takes the form of learning symptom management skills, such as adjusting to shifting mobility or coming up with efficient ways to deal with exhaustion. These accomplishments focus on regaining a sense of agency and control over one's life in addition to lessening the effects of multiple sclerosis.

The victories go beyond the person and include the group efforts of friends, family, and medical professionals. The triumphs achieved in controlling multiple sclerosis underscore the significance of a cohesive group that unites to surmount obstacles. The idea that no one is alone in their journey with MS is reinforced by the collective triumph of perseverance displayed in the face of hardship.

Furthermore, overcoming hardship frequently entails shattering prejudices about people with disabilities and societal restrictions. MS fighters turn into activists, dispelling myths about what it means to be a chronic illness sufferer. By sharing their experiences, they challenge preconceived ideas about what it means to be capable and highlight the richness of life that can be had even in the face of MS's obstacles.

A universal lesson that surpasses the particulars of every person's journey can be found in the magnificent tapestry of triumphs over adversity: the human spirit is unbreakable. These tales serve as inspiration for not only MS patients but also for anybody experiencing hardships since they show that success is not only attainable but certain when faced with resiliency, tenacity, and a caring network.

Inspirational Words from MS Proponents

Advocates are vital in the field of Multiple Sclerosis (MS) because they not only increase awareness but also offer inspirational ideas that uplift people with MS as well as the general public. These champions, who are frequently people who have personally experienced the difficulties posed by MS, share their thoughts, experiences, and information to inspire optimism and promote constructive change.

The guiding concepts of MS activists' motivational speeches are resilience, empowerment, and the conviction that a happy life is still achievable despite the obstacles presented by the illness. The significance of self-advocacy is emphasized by advocates, who exhort people with MS to actively engage in their healthcare process, consider available treatments, and make well-informed decisions.

The transformational power of thinking is a frequent element in the motivational insights shared by MS advocates. Proponents frequently discuss how developing an optimistic and flexible mindset has helped them manage the uncertainties associated with multiple sclerosis. They emphasize the significance of concentrating on what can be accomplished rather than dwelling on what cannot be accomplished, and how this change in outlook can significantly improve quality of life.

Moreover, MS activists act as links between the general public and the MS community. By presenting personal accounts and experiences, advocates humanize the condition and show that MS is not a single definition of a person but rather one component of a complex identity. They debunk myths and stereotypes about MS through writing, public speaking, and other outreach initiatives.

Motivational insights also include the promotion of research and developments in the treatment of multiple sclerosis. Proponents frequently stress the significance of keeping up with the most recent advancements, taking part in clinical trials, and endorsing projects that advance our understanding of MS. This proactive stance helps those who are directly impacted by MS and also advances our collective efforts to combat the illness.

Essentially, the inspirational words of wisdom from MS advocates act as beacons, shedding light on pathways of resiliency, self-determination, and optimism for individuals navigating the challenges of the disease. Their voices collectively convey a message that MS does not define one's capabilities and that, with perseverance and advocacy, a meaningful and fulfilling life is not only possible but completely achievable.

Developing Future Hope and Resilience

Building resilience and fostering hope for the future are not simply goals in the difficult world of living with Multiple Sclerosis (MS); they are vital elements of a comprehensive approach to well-being. With its fluctuating symptoms and unpredictable nature, multiple sclerosis (MS) necessitates not just physical adaptation but also a strong mental and emotional resilience that empowers people to face each day with bravery and hope.

Creating coping mechanisms that enable people to manage the uncertainties associated with multiple sclerosis (MS) is a key component of building resilience. Some examples of these mechanisms include practicing mindfulness, getting help from mental health providers, or participating in activities that enhance emotional health. Instead of eliminating obstacles, resilience is about cultivating the inner fortitude to face them head-on and overcome failures.

The development of a support system is a crucial component of resilience building. A strong support network, whether it consists of friends, family, MS patients, or medical professionals, offers a basis for both practical and emotional help. A supportive network that shares stories, struggles, and victories helps people feel like they belong and that they are not alone in their MS journey.

Developing hope for the future is seeing past the immediate obstacles that MS presents. It includes establishing reasonable objectives, pursuing interests, and staying purposeful. People who have multiple sclerosis (MS) frequently draw motivation from the achievements of those who have effectively managed the condition's complications, which strengthens their conviction that a happy life is still attainable despite the challenges.

Furthermore, campaigns for advocacy and awareness are entwined with hopes for the future. People with MS who actively engage in advocacy work add to a larger movement aimed at enhancing knowledge, resources, and treatment choices. In addition to empowering the individual advocate, this active participation raises hopes for positive change within the MS community as a whole.

The inspiring tales of people with multiple sclerosis serve as a great thread in the larger fabric of fostering future hope and resilience. They show that it is possible to not only survive but also thrive in the face of a chronic and unpredictable ailment. People with MS create a road forward through resiliency and hope, showing the rest of the world that the future is determined by the opportunities that lie ahead rather than by the obstacles of the present.

www.ingramcontent.com/pod-product-compliance
Lightning Source LLC
Chambersburg PA
CBHW071600270726
48661CB00017B/258